KEYS TO FERTILITY

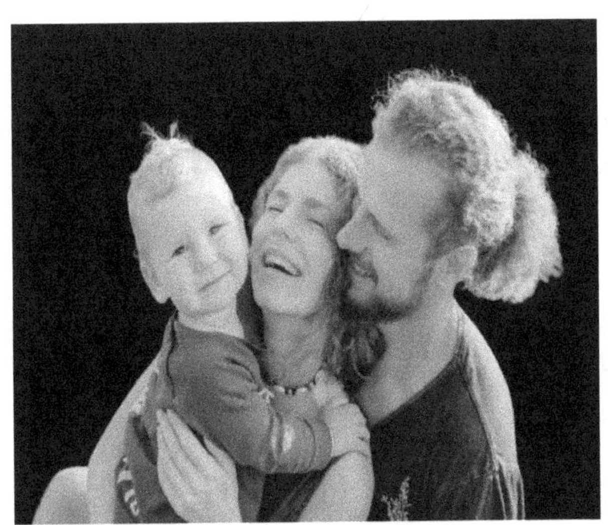

A lucid guide to improving your Fertility status, reproductive health, birth control and end miscarriage for men and women.

By Ella Samuel

TABLE OF CONTENTS

- Lifestyle and dietary changes to support a healthy pregnancy

- Medical interventions and treatments to prevent miscarriage

Chapter 7: Assisted Reproductive Technologies and Miscarriage

- The role of assisted reproductive technologies (ART) in fertility treatments

- The potential risks and success rates of ART in relation to miscarriage

- Counseling and support for couples undergoing ART

Unlocking the keys to fertility and ending the heartbreak of miscarriage is a deeply personal and significant journey. For those who long for the joy of conceiving and carrying a child to term, the challenges and disappointment can be agonizing. Countless individuals and couples find themselves seeking answers, solutions, and ultimately, hope.

In this book, we delve into the intricate complexities of fertility and the pain of miscarriage, offering you a comprehensive guide to understanding the underlying causes and discovering effective strategies to overcome these obstacles. Whether you are just beginning your fertility journey or have experienced the heartache of recurrent miscarriages, this book aims to provide you with the knowledge, support, and guidance you need to unlock your fertility and end the cycle of loss.

Chapter by chapter, we will explore the science behind fertility, deciphering the mysteries of conception, and navigating the labyrinth of causes that lead to infertility. We will break down the various factors that may contribute to miscarriage and empower you with practical steps to minimize these risks. From lifestyle changes to medical interventions, we leave no stone unturned in our pursuit of solutions.

But this book is not just about the physical aspects of fertility and miscarriage; it delves deep into the emotional and mental toll that these challenges can take.

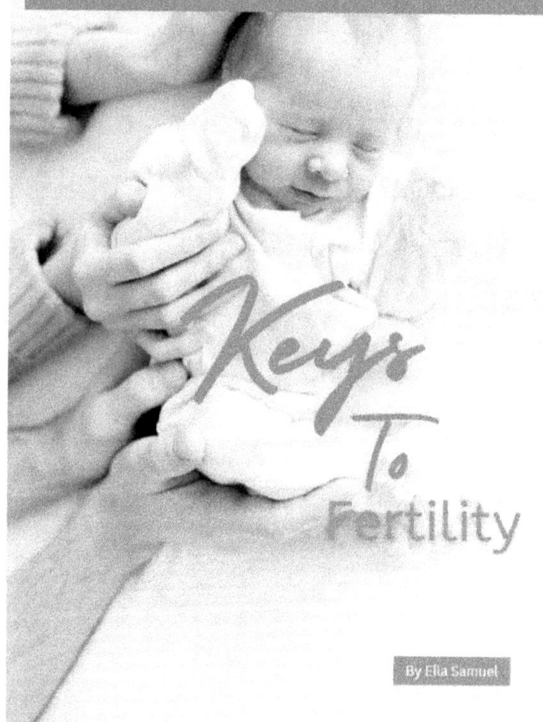

A lucid guide to improving your Fertility status, reproductive health, birth control and end miscarriage for men and women
Keys
To
Fertility
By Ella Samuel

CHAPTER 1

Understanding Fertility and Miscarriage

-Infertility is defined as the inability to conceive after a year of regular, unprotected intercourse for couples under the age of 35, or after six months for couples over the age of 35. There are various causes of infertility, and it is often a multifactorial condition. Some common causes include:

1. Hormonal imbalances: Hormonal imbalances can disrupt the delicate balance required for successful conception. Conditions such as polycystic ovary syndrome

(PCOS) and thyroid disorders can affect hormone production and ovulation.

2. Structural abnormalities: Structural abnormalities in the reproductive organs, such as blocked fallopian tubes or uterine fibroids, can interfere with the fertilization process or implantation.

3. Ovulation disorders: Ovulation disorders, where the ovaries do not release eggs regularly or at all, can significantly impact fertility. Common examples include hypothalamic amenorrhea, where the hypothalamus does not release sufficient hormones to stimulate ovulation, and premature

ovarian failure, where the ovaries stop functioning before the age of 40.

4. Endometriosis: When endometriosis occurs, the uterine lining develops outside of the organ. This abnormal tissue growth can cause chronic inflammation, scarring, and adhesions, leading to infertility.

5. Male factor infertility: Infertility is not solely a female issue; male factor infertility contributes to approximately 40% of infertility cases. Causes of male infertility include low sperm count, poor sperm quality, and structural abnormalities in the reproductive organs.

-Understanding the basics of the reproductive system is crucial in comprehending fertility and the factors that may affect it. The uterus, fallopian tubes, vagina, and ovaries make up the female reproductive system. Each month, one of the ovaries releases an egg, which then travels down the fallopian tube, where it may be fertilized by sperm. If fertilization occurs, the fertilized egg implants itself into the uterus, where it develops into a fetus. If fertilization does not occur, the lining of the uterus is shed during menstruation.

The male reproductive system includes the testes, which

produce sperm, and the penis, which delivers sperm into the female reproductive system.

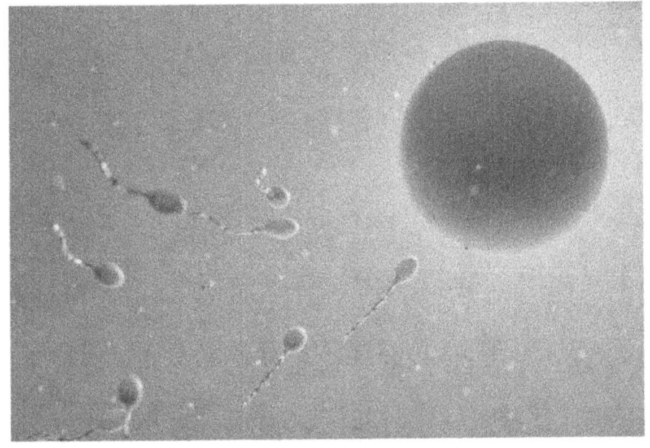

-A miscarriage occurs when a pregnancy ends before the 20th week; it is also referred to as a spontaneous abortion. Common causes of miscarriage include:

1. Chromosomal abnormalities: The most common cause of

miscarriage is chromosomal abnormalities in the fetus. These abnormalities usually occur by chance during the formation of sperm or egg, resulting in an embryo with an abnormal number of chromosomes.

2. Hormonal imbalances: Hormonal imbalances, such as low levels of progesterone, can affect the uterus's ability to support a pregnancy and can increase the risk of miscarriage.

3. Uterine abnormalities: Structural abnormalities in the uterus, such as uterine fibroids, polyps, or septum, can disrupt the implantation process and lead to miscarriage.

4. Infections: Certain infections, such as bacterial vaginosis, urinary tract infections, or sexually transmitted infections, can increase the risk of miscarriage.

5. Immunological factors: In some cases, the immune system may recognize the embryo as foreign and mount an immune response, leading to miscarriage.

6. Chronic health conditions: Chronic health conditions, such as diabetes, thyroid disorders, or autoimmune disorders, can increase the risk of miscarriage.

7. Lifestyle factors: Factors such as advanced maternal age, smoking, alcohol consumption,

drug abuse, and obesity can also increase the risk of miscarriage.

Understanding the causes and factors that contribute to infertility and miscarriage is the first step towards finding effective solutions and support. In the subsequent chapters, we will delve deeper into each aspect, providing you with insights, strategies, and resources to navigate your fertility journey.

CHAPTER 2

Preparing the Body for Fertility

The journey towards achieving fertility begins with preparing the body for reproduction. Making certain lifestyle changes, adopting a nutritious diet, incorporating exercise, and reaching a healthy weight can significantly improve reproductive health and enhance fertility.

- Lifestyle Changes: Lifestyle factors play a crucial role in fertility. Several habits and behaviors can negatively impact fertility, such as smoking, excessive alcohol consumption, drug use, and high levels of stress. Quitting smoking and limiting alcohol and drug use can improve fertility outcomes. Additionally, managing stress through techniques like meditation, yoga, or counseling can help regulate hormonal balance and promote optimal reproductive health.

- Nutrition and Fertility: The role of nutrition in fertility cannot be overstated. A healthy diet rich in fruits, vegetables, whole grains, lean proteins, and healthy fats can positively impact fertility outcomes. Key nutrients that support reproductive health include folate, iron, zinc, vitamin D, and omega-3 fatty acids. Avoiding processed foods, sugary beverages, and excessive caffeine consumption is also recommended.

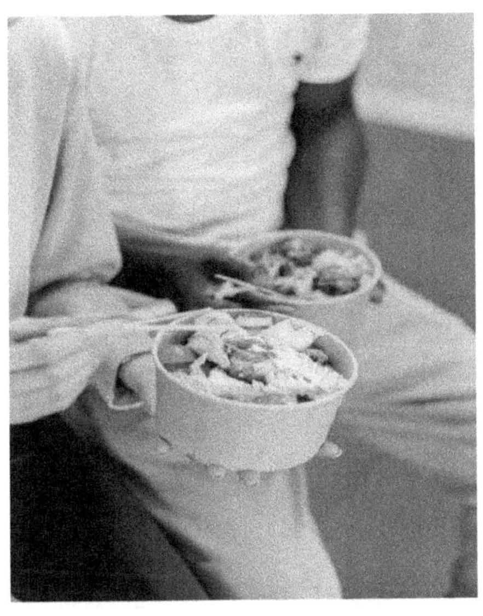

- Exercise and Reproductive Health: Regular exercise has numerous benefits for reproductive health. It can help regulate hormones, improve blood flow to the reproductive

organs, maintain a healthy

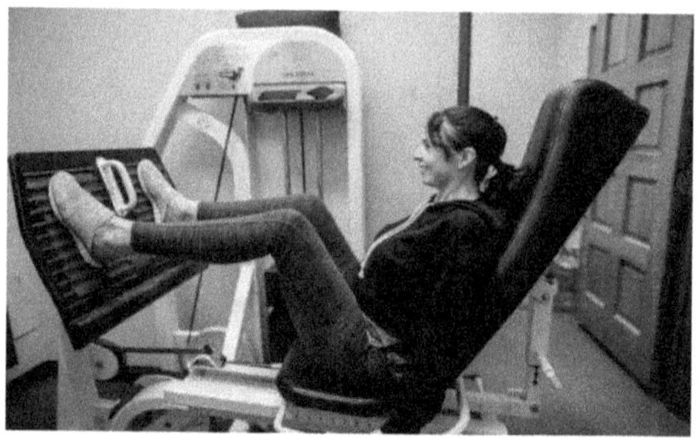

weight, and reduce the risk of chronic conditions that may affect fertility. However, it is essential to strike a balance as excessive exercise or high-intensity workouts can actually have a negative impact on fertility. Aim for moderate-intensity exercise, such as brisk walking, swimming, or cycling, for at least 30 minutes most days of the week.

- Getting to a Healthy Weight: Achieving a healthy weight is crucial for optimizing fertility. Both being underweight and overweight can disrupt hormone production and menstrual cycles, making it more challenging to conceive. If you are underweight, gaining weight through a balanced diet and regular exercise can improve fertility. If you are overweight or obese, losing weight through a combination of diet and exercise can enhance fertility outcomes.

Consulting with a healthcare professional specializing in reproductive health can provide personalized recommendations based on your specific circumstances and needs. They can assess your current health, identify potential barriers to fertility, and develop a tailored plan to prepare your body for pregnancy.

In the next chapter, we will delve into the intricacies of the menstrual cycle and how understanding your cycle can empower you to maximize your fertility potential.

Optimizing fertility naturally

 Chapter 3 of "Optimizing Fertility Naturally" delves into the crucial aspects of understanding the menstrual cycle, tracking ovulation and fertile days, and exploring natural remedies and techniques for boosting fertility.

The menstrual cycle is the monthly hormonal cycle that prepares a woman's body for possible pregnancy. It typically lasts about 28 days, although variations are common. Understanding the menstrual cycle is essential for optimizing fertility naturally.

The first phase of the menstrual cycle is called the follicular phase, which begins on the first day of menstruation. During this phase, the body prepares an egg for release. The second phase, the ovulatory phase, occurs around day 14 of the cycle when the mature egg is released from the ovary. The final phase, the luteal phase, begins after ovulation and lasts until the start of the next menstrual cycle.

Tracking ovulation and fertile days is crucial when trying to conceive. Ovulation usually occurs about 14 days before the start of the next menstruation. Several methods can help identify ovulation, such as tracking basal body temperature, observing changes in cervical mucus, and using ovulation predictor kits. By understanding their menstrual cycle and identifying the fertile days, couples can time intercourse to increase the chances of conception.

Natural remedies and techniques can be used to boost fertility. Here are some examples:

1. Healthy lifestyle choices: Maintaining a healthy weight, exercising regularly, and managing stress can positively impact fertility. Obesity and excessive exercise can disrupt hormonal balance, while stress

can interfere with ovulation and menstrual regularity.

2. Balanced diet: A nutrient-rich diet can support reproductive health. Including a variety of fruits, vegetables, whole grains, lean proteins, and healthy fats can provide essential vitamins and minerals. Foods rich in antioxidants, such as berries, leafy greens, and nuts, can also promote fertility.

3. Herbal remedies: Certain herbs have been traditionally used to support fertility. Examples include chaste berry (Vitex agnus-castus), red raspberry leaf, maca root, and Dong Quai. These herbs are believed to promote hormonal

balance and regulate the menstrual cycle. Before utilizing herbal medicines, it's crucial to speak with a healthcare provider because they can have contraindications or interfere with pharmaceuticals.

4. Acupuncture: This ancient Chinese therapy involves the insertion of thin needles into specific points on the body to promote balance and energy flow. Acupuncture can be used to address various fertility issues, such as hormonal imbalances, ovarian dysfunction, and stress.

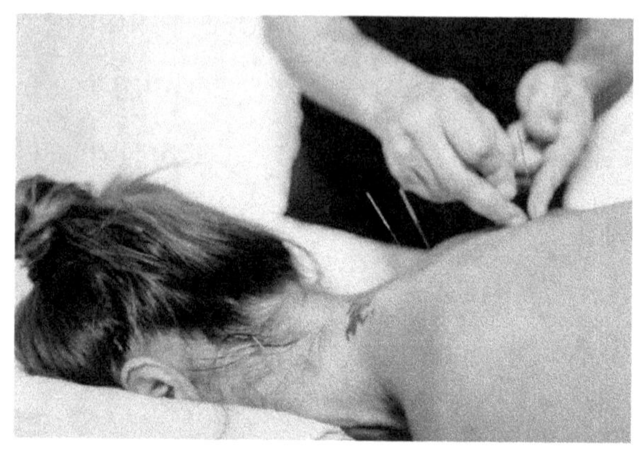

5. Stress management techniques: Chronic stress can negatively impact fertility. Techniques such as meditation, yoga, mindfulness, and deep breathing exercises can help reduce stress levels, promote relaxation, and improve overall well-being.

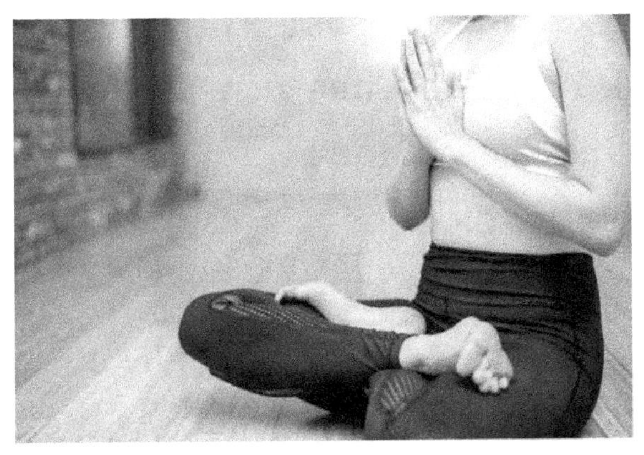

6. Natural supplements: Certain supplements have been suggested to support fertility. Examples include CoQ10, omega-3 fatty acids, vitamin D, and fertility-specific multivitamins. It is important to consult with a healthcare professional before starting any supplements, as they may have interactions or contraindications.

7. Avoiding toxins: Exposure to toxins in the environment, such as pesticides, heavy metals, and chemicals found in certain household products, can interfere with fertility. It is important to minimize exposure to these toxins and choose natural and organic alternatives whenever possible.

Optimizing fertility naturally involves understanding the menstrual cycle, tracking ovulation and fertile days, and implementing natural remedies and techniques. By incorporating these practices into their lifestyle, couples can enhance their fertility and increase their chances of conceiving.

CHAPTER 4

Seeking Medical Help for Fertility Challenges

Seeking professional help for fertility challenges is an important step for many couples who have been trying to conceive without success. While it is natural for conception to take some time, there are certain factors that may indicate the need for medical intervention. Here are some considerations for when to seek professional help:

1. Age: Women age 35 and older may want to seek fertility help earlier, as fertility declines with age. It is recommended to

consult a fertility specialist if conception has not occurred after six months of regular, unprotected intercourse for women over 35.

2. Irregular periods: Women who have irregular menstrual cycles may have difficulty predicting ovulation or have hormonal imbalances that affect their fertility. If periods are consistently irregular or absent, medical intervention can help identify and treat these underlying issues.

3. Known reproductive health conditions: Women with known reproductive health conditions, such as polycystic ovary syndrome (PCOS),

endometriosis, or pelvic inflammatory disease (PID), may have fertility challenges. Consulting with a fertility specialist can help manage these conditions and optimize the chances of conception.

4. Male factor infertility: Infertility is not solely a female issue. Male factor infertility, such as low sperm count or poor sperm quality, can also contribute to difficulties conceiving. If a couple has been trying to conceive for a year without success, it is recommended for both partners to undergo fertility testing.

5. Previous pregnancy complications: Couples who

have experienced recurrent miscarriages or pregnancy complications may benefit from seeking help sooner rather than later. Fertility specialists can evaluate the underlying causes and develop a treatment plan to improve chances of a successful pregnancy.

-Once professional help is sought, there are various fertility treatments and procedures that may be recommended based on the specific circumstances. Here are some common options:

1. Ovulation induction: This involves the use of medications, such as clomiphene citrate or letrozole, to stimulate ovulation

in women who are not ovulating regularly.

2. Intrauterine insemination (IUI): In this procedure, washed and concentrated sperm are directly placed into the uterus during the fertile window, increasing the chances of successful fertilization.

3. In vitro fertilization (IVF): IVF involves the retrieval of eggs and fertilization with sperm in a laboratory setting. The resulting embryos are then transferred to the uterus. IVF is often recommended for couples with severe male factor infertility, blocked fallopian tubes, or other fertility issues.

4. Assisted reproductive technologies (ART): ART includes various advanced techniques that can be used alongside IVF, such as intracytoplasmic sperm injection (ICSI), where a single sperm is injected directly into an egg. Other ART options include preimplantation genetic testing (PGT) to screen embryos for chromosomal abnormalities before transfer.

5. Donor sperm or eggs: In cases where there are severe male or female fertility issues, using donor sperm or eggs may be an option. This involves using sperm or eggs from a third-party donor for fertilization.

It's important to note that each couple's fertility journey is unique, and the recommended treatments and procedures may vary depending on the individual circumstances. Fertility specialists will work closely with couples to determine the best course of action.

-In addition to conventional fertility treatments, some couples may also choose to explore 4alternative and complementary therapies. These therapies are often used alongside medical interventions to support overall fertility and well-being. Some examples include:

1. Acupuncture: Acupuncture
has been used for centuries to
promote fertility and
reproductive health. It is
believed to help regulate
hormones, improve blood flow
to the reproductive organs, and
reduce stress.

2. Herbal medicine: Herbal
remedies and supplements, such
as chaste berry (Vitex), maca
root, and red raspberry leaf, are
sometimes used to support
hormonal balance and enhance
fertility. It is important to consult
with a qualified herbalist or
healthcare provider before using
any herbal remedies, as they
may interact with medications or
have contraindications.

3. Mind-body therapies: Techniques such as meditation, yoga, and mindfulness can help reduce stress and promote relaxation, which in turn may positively impact fertility.

4. Nutritional and lifestyle modifications: Making dietary and lifestyle changes can have a significant impact on fertility. Following a balanced diet, reducing alcohol and caffeine intake, quitting smoking, and managing stress can improve overall reproductive health.

It is important for couples considering alternative or complementary therapies to discuss these options with their healthcare provider or a qualified specialist. They can provide guidance and help determine which therapies may be suitable and safe for each individual.

In conclusion, seeking professional help for fertility challenges is a crucial step for couples struggling to conceive. Fertility treatments and procedures, along with alternative and complementary therapies, can provide options and support in the journey towards parenthood. Each couple's path is unique, and it is important to work closely with healthcare.

CHAPTER 5

Emotional and Mental Well-being in the Fertility Journey

-Coping with the stress and emotional impact of infertility

The fertility journey can be emotionally and mentally challenging for individuals and couples. Dealing with the stress, disappointment, and grief associated with infertility requires a strong emotional support system and effective coping mechanisms. Here are some strategies for coping with the emotional impact of infertility:

1. Acknowledge and express emotions: It is important to

allow yourself to feel and express your emotions, whether it be sadness, anger, frustration, or fear. Recognize that it is normal to experience a range of emotions and give yourself permission to express them in healthy ways.

2. Seek support: Utilize your support system by confiding in friends, family, or a therapist who can provide a caring and non-judgmental space for you to share your feelings. Joining a support group for individuals or couples going through infertility can also be helpful in providing a sense of community and understanding.

3. Self care: Take care of your physical, emotional, and mental needs by engaging in self-care. Take part in enjoyable and soothing activities, such hobbies, meditation, physical activity, or time spent in nature. Make self-care activities that feed your body, mind, and spirit a priority.

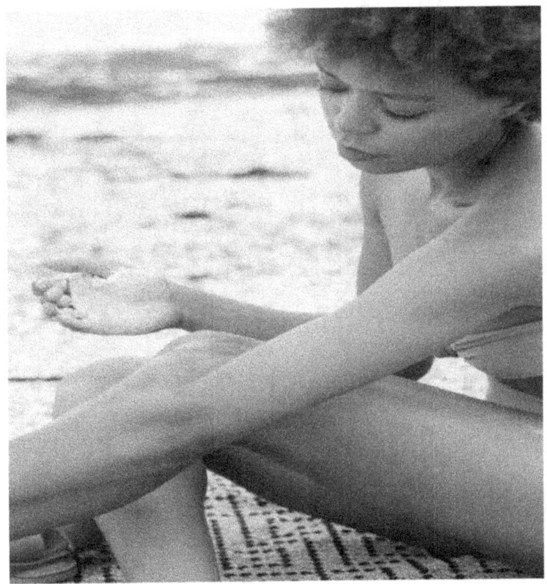

4. Set boundaries: It's important to set boundaries with others, especially when it comes to discussions and questions about your fertility journey. Protecting your emotional well-being and privacy is crucial, and it is perfectly acceptable to let others know what topics or questions are off-limits.

5. Practice stress management techniques: Find healthy and effective ways to manage stress, such as deep breathing exercises, meditation, yoga, or engaging in activities that help you relax and unwind. Regularly practicing stress management techniques can help reduce

anxiety and promote emotional well-being.

In addition to coping with the emotional impact of infertility, it is important to actively nurture and enhance emotional well-being. Here are some strategies for promoting emotional well-being during the fertility journey:

1. Educate yourself: Understanding the various aspects of fertility, fertility treatments, and available options can help empower you and alleviate feelings of uncertainty and helplessness. Stay informed and seek out

reputable resources to educate yourself on the fertility journey.

2. Communicate with your partner: Open and honest communication with your partner is essential. Share your thoughts, feelings, and concerns with each other and actively work together as a team. Regularly check in with each other and discuss how you both are coping with the fertility journey and any adjustments that may need to be made.

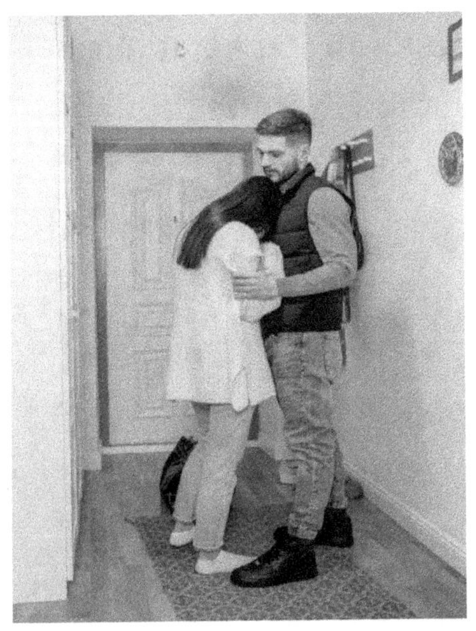

3. Focus on the present moment: It's easy to get caught up in the future and the uncertainty of the fertility journey. Remain mindful and concentrate on the here and now. Engage in activities that bring you joy and fulfillment in the here and now.

4. Set realistic expectations: Understand that the fertility journey can be unpredictable and may involve setbacks and challenges. Setting realistic expectations can help manage disappointment and maintain a positive outlook. Remember that everyone's journey is unique, and there is no one-size-fits-all timeline or outcome.

5. Seek professional help: If you find that the emotional toll of infertility becomes overwhelming or starts to affect your daily life, consider reaching out to a mental health professional who specializes in fertility-related issues. They can provide support, guidance, and

coping strategies tailored to your specific needs.

Support systems and resources

Building a strong support system and utilizing available resources can provide valuable emotional support throughout the fertility journey. Here are some support systems and resources to consider:

1. Friends and family: Lean on your loved ones for emotional support. Share your feelings with trusted friends and family members who can provide empathy, understanding, and encouragement.

2. Support groups: Joining a support group specifically for

individuals or couples going through infertility can be incredibly beneficial. These groups provide a safe space to share experiences, gain insights from others who are going through similar challenges, and offer support and encouragement.

3. Online communities and forums: Online communities and forums dedicated to infertility can provide a sense of community and connection. They offer a platform to connect with others, share experiences, and seek advice and support.

4. Fertility clinics and healthcare providers: Fertility clinics often have resources and support

services available, including counseling, support groups, and educational materials. Additionally, healthcare providers who specialize in fertility can offer guidance and support throughout the fertility journey.

5. Mental health professionals: Consider seeking support from mental health professionals who specialize in infertility. Therapists or counselors can provide emotional support, help navigate the emotional challenges of infertility, and offer coping strategies.

6. Books and educational resources: There are a variety of books, blogs, and articles

available that provide information and support for individuals and couples experiencing infertility. These resources can offer helpful insights, practical tips, and personal stories of others going through similar journeys.

Remember, it's important to personalize your support system and resources to meet your specific needs. Find what works best for you and don't hesitate to reach out for support when needed. The fertility journey can be emotionally taxing, but with the right support and resources, you can navigate through it with strength and resilience.

CHAPTER 6

Preventing Miscarriage and Supporting Pregnancy

Understanding the risk factors for miscarriage:

Miscarriage, also known as spontaneous abortion, is the loss of a pregnancy before the fetus is able to survive outside the womb. It is estimated that about 10-20% of known pregnancies end in miscarriage, with the majority occurring within the first trimester.

While a miscarriage can occur for various reasons, there are certain risk factors that can increase the likelihood of it happening. Some common risk factors include:

1. Advanced maternal age: Women who are older than 35 are at a higher risk of miscarriage compared to younger women.

2. Previous miscarriage: Women who have had one or more previous miscarriages are at an increased risk of experiencing another miscarriage.

3. Certain medical conditions: Conditions such as diabetes, thyroid disorders, polycystic ovary syndrome (PCOS), and autoimmune disorders can increase the risk of miscarriage.

4. Genetic abnormalities: Fetuses with chromosomal abnormalities, such as Down syndrome, are more likely to be miscarried.

5. Uterine abnormalities: Structural issues with the uterus, such as fibroids or a septate uterus, can increase the risk of miscarriage.

6. Hormonal imbalances: Low levels of progesterone, a hormone necessary for sustaining a pregnancy, can increase the risk of miscarriage.

Lifestyle and dietary changes to support a healthy pregnancy:

Making certain lifestyle and dietary changes can help support a healthy pregnancy and reduce the risk of miscarriage. Here are some recommendations:

1. Maintain a healthy weight: Being underweight or overweight can increase the risk of miscarriage. It is important to aim for a healthy weight before getting pregnant and to continue making healthy choices throughout pregnancy.

2. Eat a balanced diet: Focus on consuming a variety of nutrient-dense foods, including fruits, vegetables, lean proteins, whole grains, and healthy fats. Avoid processed foods, excessive caffeine, and alcohol. It is also important to take prenatal vitamins to ensure adequate

nutrient intake, particularly folic
acid, which helps prevent certain
birth defects.

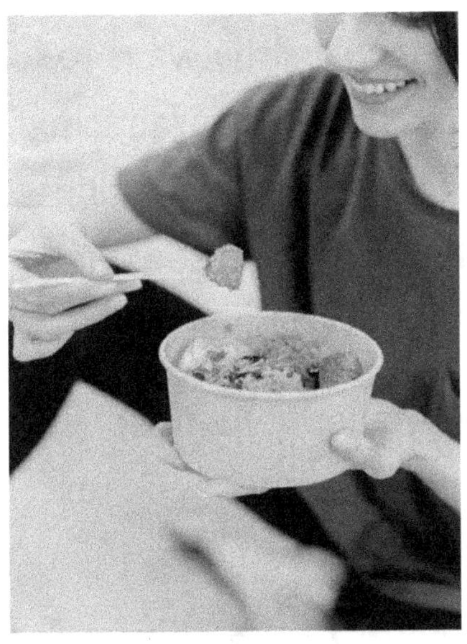

3. Avoid harmful substances:
Smoking, drug use, and excessive
alcohol consumption are all
associated with an increased risk
of miscarriage. It is important to

avoid these substances before and during pregnancy.

4. Manage stress: High levels of stress can impact pregnancy outcomes. Find healthy ways to manage stress, such as practicing relaxation techniques, engaging in physical activity, and seeking support from loved ones.

5. Exercise regularly: Regular physical activity is beneficial for overall health and can help support a healthy pregnancy. Before beginning or maintaining an exercise regimen while pregnant, it's crucial to speak with a healthcare provider.

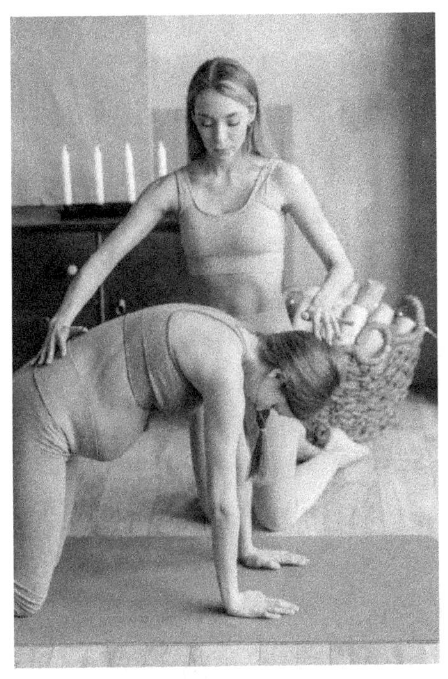

Medical interventions and treatments to prevent miscarriage:

In some cases, medical interventions and treatments may be recommended to prevent a miscarriage or reduce the risk. These may include:

1. Progesterone supplementation: If low progesterone levels are identified as a risk factor, progesterone supplementation may be prescribed to support the pregnancy.

2. Cervical cerclage: In cases where there is a weakness in the cervix or a history of mid-trimester miscarriage, a cervical cerclage may be performed. This is a procedure in which a stitch is placed around the cervix to provide support and help prevent miscarriage.

3. Lifestyle modifications: If certain lifestyle factors, such as smoking, excessive alcohol consumption, or substance abuse, are identified as risk factors, counseling and support may be provided to help the individual make necessary changes.

4. Genetic testing: If recurrent miscarriages are experienced, genetic testing may be recommended to identify any underlying genetic abnormalities that could be contributing to the miscarriages. Depending on the results, further treatments or interventions may be suggested.

It is important to understand that not all miscarriages can be prevented, and sometimes they occur due to factors that are beyond anyone's control. However, by understanding the risk factors, making appropriate lifestyle and dietary changes, and seeking medical interventions when necessary, it is possible to reduce the risk of miscarriage and support a healthy pregnancy. For individualized counsel and direction, speaking with a healthcare professional is always advised.

CHAPTER 7

Assisted Reproductive Technologies and Miscarriage

-Assisted reproductive technologies (ART) have revolutionized the field of fertility treatments and have provided hope for countless couples struggling with infertility. ART includes a range of procedures such as in vitro fertilization (IVF), intracytoplasmic sperm injection (ICSI), and preimplantation genetic testing (PGT), among others.

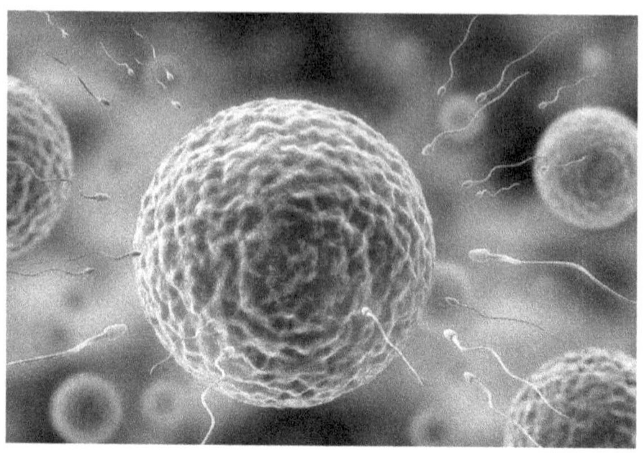

While ART has significantly increased the chances of pregnancy and live birth for couples, it is important to understand the potential risks of these treatments in relation to miscarriage. Miscarriage after ART is a possibility, although the exact rates vary depending on factors such as the woman's age, underlying fertility issues, and the specific procedures used.

-Some research suggests that the risk of miscarriage after IVF is slightly higher than that of natural conceptions. However, it is essential to interpret these findings cautiously, as there are other factors to consider. For example, couples undergoing ART often face more age-related infertility concerns or genetic abnormalities in embryos, which can independently increase the risk of miscarriage.

-Counseling and pre-treatment discussions are crucial components of the ART process. Healthcare providers should inform couples about the risks and success rates associated with ART, as well as the potential emotional and psychological challenges they may face. This allows couples to make informed decisions and set realistic expectations.

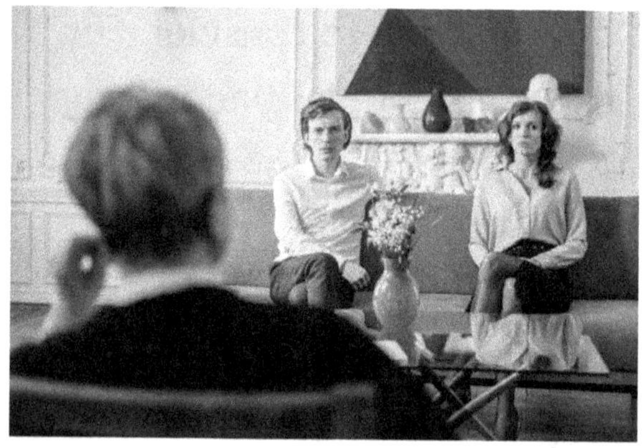

In cases where couples have experienced previous miscarriages, additional counseling and support may be necessary. This can help them process their emotions, address any concerns or fears they may have, and make decisions about moving forward with ART.

Support groups and counseling services specifically for couples undergoing ART can be beneficial. These provide a safe space for sharing experiences, seeking advice, and receiving emotional support from others who are going through similar challenges. Mental health professionals trained in infertility and miscarriage can also provide individual counseling to help couples cope with the emotional toll of miscarriage and further treatment.

It is important to note that success rates with ART have improved over the years, and many couples are ultimately able to conceive and have a healthy pregnancy. However, it is equally important to acknowledge that there are no guarantees, and miscarriage can still occur. Providing comprehensive counseling and support throughout the ART process can help couples navigate the emotional rollercoaster and make decisions that are right for them.

CHAPTER 8

Other Factors Affecting Fertility and Miscarriage

Age and Its Impact on Fertility and Miscarriage:

Age is a significant factor that affects both fertility and the risk of miscarriage. Women are born with a finite number of eggs, and as they age, the quantity and quality of those eggs decline. This decline in fertility becomes more significant after the age of 35 and accelerates after 40.

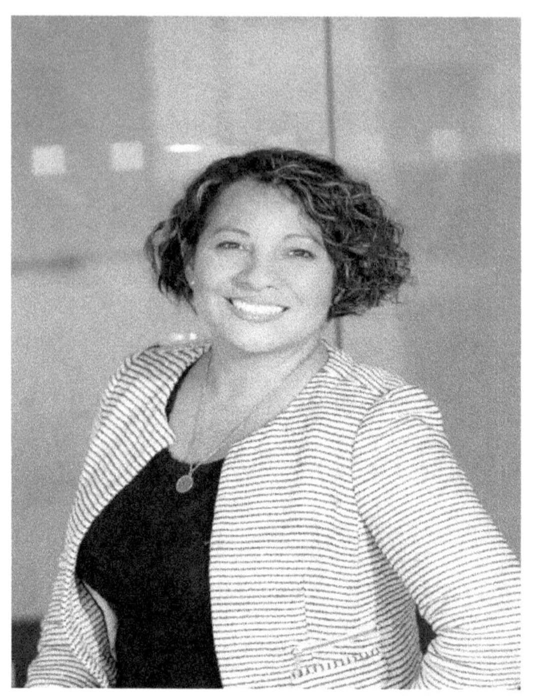

Advanced maternal age is associated with a higher risk of chromosome abnormalities in embryos, which can lead to miscarriage or birth defects. Additionally, older women may have higher rates of underlying health conditions, such as diabetes or hypertension, which can also increase the risk of miscarriage.

Environmental Factors and Their Effects on Reproductive Health:

Exposure to certain environmental factors can have negative effects on reproductive health and increase the risk of miscarriage. These factors can include:

1. Chemical exposure: Exposure to toxic chemicals, such as pesticides, heavy metals, solvents, and pollutants, can impact reproductive health. Prolonged exposure to these substances can affect both male

and female fertility and increase the risk of miscarriage.

2. Radiation: High levels of radiation exposure, such as from medical procedures or radiation therapy, can harm reproductive organs and lead to infertility or an increased risk of miscarriage.

3. Lifestyle factors: Certain lifestyle choices, such as smoking, excessive alcohol consumption, and illicit drug use, can negatively impact fertility and increase the risk of miscarriage.

4. Stress: Chronic stress can disrupt hormonal balance and impact reproductive function. While there is no direct causal

link between stress and miscarriage, it is believed that high-stress levels can increase the risk.

Genetic Factors and Testing for Potential Fertility Issues:

Genetic factors can play a role in fertility issues and the risk of miscarriage. Genetic testing can help identify potential underlying issues and inform treatment decisions. Some genetic factors to consider include:

1. Chromosomal abnormalities: Structural or numerical abnormalities in the chromosomes can increase the risk of miscarriage. Testing for

chromosomal abnormalities in both partners can help determine if additional interventions, such as preimplantation genetic testing, are needed during fertility treatments.

2. Genetic disorders: Certain inherited genetic disorders, such as cystic fibrosis or sickle cell disease, can affect fertility and increase the risk of miscarriage. Genetic testing can identify carriers of these disorders and inform reproductive decisions.

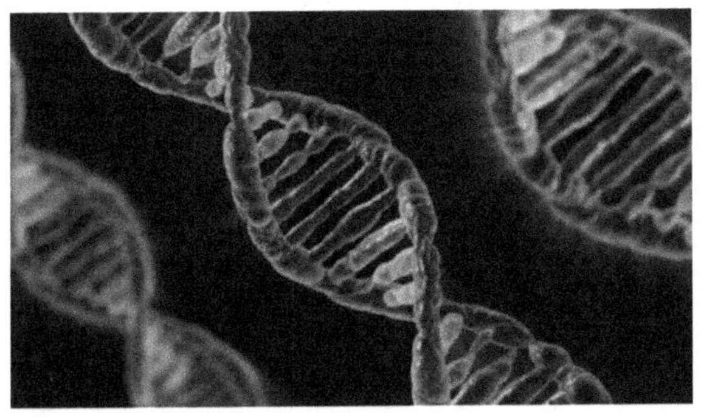

3. Genetic carrier screening: Screening tests, such as carrier screening, can identify individuals who carry genetic mutations that could be passed on to their offspring. This information can help couples make informed decisions about family planning options and may also influence the choice of fertility treatments.

In summary, age, environmental factors, and genetic factors can all play a role in fertility and the risk of miscarriage. Understanding these factors and seeking appropriate testing and interventions can help individuals and couples make informed decisions and improve their chances of a successful pregnancy. It is recommended to consult with healthcare professionals with expertise in fertility and reproductive health to discuss individual circumstances and explore potential strategies for addressing these factors.

CHAPTER 9

Navigating the Emotional Rollercoaster of Infertility and Miscarriage

Dealing with grief and loss:

Dealing with the emotional impact of infertility and miscarriage can be incredibly challenging. It is important to acknowledge and process the grief and loss that comes with these experiences. Here are some strategies for navigating the emotional rollercoaster:

1. Give yourself permission to feel and express your feelings as you grieve. It is normal to experience a range of emotions, including sadness, anger,

frustration, and guilt. Give yourself permission to mourn in your own time and manner.

2. Seek support: Reach out to your support system, whether it be your partner, family, friends, or a support group. Having someone to talk to and lean on can provide comfort and understanding.

3. Consider counseling: Professional counseling can be beneficial in helping you process your emotions and develop coping strategies. A therapist who specializes in infertility and pregnancy loss can provide guidance and support.

4.Observe self-care: Make self-care a priority by doing things that make you happy and calm. This could include exercise, practicing mindfulness or meditation, seeking out hobbies, or pampering yourself with self-care rituals.

Communication and support within relationships:

Infertility and miscarriage can strain relationships, but open communication and support are crucial for navigating these challenges together. These are a few methods for helping one another out.

1. Share your feelings: Openly communicate your emotions and

fears with your partner. Create a safe space for both of you to express your thoughts and feelings without judgment.

2. Be empathetic: Recognize that both partners may experience different emotions and cope in different ways. Try to empathize with each other's perspectives and validate each other's feelings.

3. Seek professional help if needed: If the emotional toll becomes too overwhelming, consider seeking couples counseling or therapy. A professional can help facilitate productive communication and provide guidance for navigating these challenges as a couple.

4. Create a support system: Connect with other couples or individuals going through similar experiences. Joining a support group or seeking online communities can provide a sense of belonging and understanding.

Having resilience and hope when faced with obstacles:

Infertility and miscarriage can be emotionally draining, but finding hope and resilience is essential for moving forward. In order to discover hope, try these strategies:

1. Educate yourself: Learn about the many available treatments and technologies. Knowledge

can empower you and give you hope for the future.

2. Focus on the present: While it's important to have hope for the future, it's also important to focus on the present moment. Engage in activities that bring you joy and fulfillment outside of your fertility journey.

3. Practice self-compassion: Be gentle with yourself and practice self-compassion. Acknowledge that you are doing the best you can and that it's okay to have bad days.

4. Explore alternative paths to parenthood: If conceiving naturally is not possible, consider exploring alternative

paths to parenthood, such as adoption or surrogacy. These options can provide a new sense of hope and possibility.

5. Stay connected with your partner :

Maintain a strong connection with your partner by nurturing your relationship and finding joy in the journey together. Remember that you are in this together, supporting each other through the highs and lows.

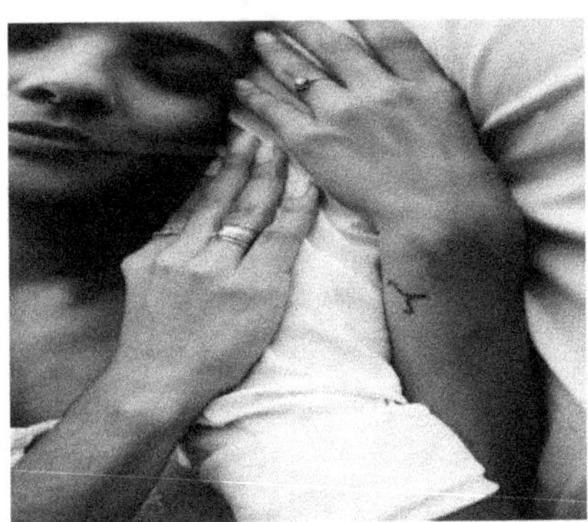

Infertility and miscarriage are emotionally challenging experiences, but with support, open communication, and resilience, it is possible to navigate the rollercoaster. Remember to be patient with yourself and seek professional help when needed. There is hope for building a family, and your journey will be unique to you.

CHAPTER 10

Moving Forward and Building a Family

Strategies for acceptance and managing expectations:

1. Reflect on your goals and values: Take the time to reflect on what building a family means to you and what values are important to you. This can help you gain clarity and focus on what truly matters to you.

2. Practice acceptance: Acceptance does not mean giving up on your dreams but rather accepting the reality of your situation. Acknowledge that your journey may be different from what you initially imagined,

and focus on finding joy and fulfillment in the path you are on.

3. Set realistic expectations: Understand that building a family may not happen overnight and may involve setbacks and challenges along the way. Set realistic expectations for yourself and be prepared for the journey to take time.

Exploring alternative paths to parenthood:

1. Adoption: Consider exploring adoption as a means of building your family. Adoption provides an opportunity to provide a loving home to a child in need

and can be a rewarding and
fulfilling path to parenthood.

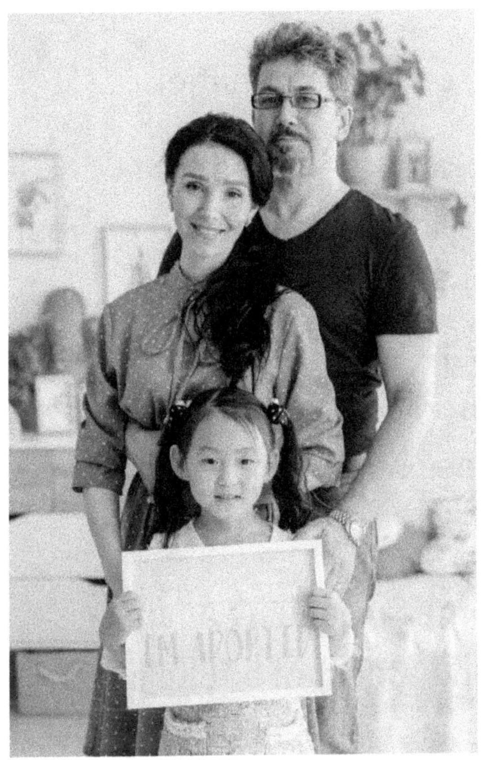

2. Surrogacy: For couples who
are unable to carry a pregnancy
to term, surrogacy can be an
option. This involves another

woman carrying and giving birth to the child on behalf of the intended parents.

3. Egg or sperm donation

4. Explore career and professional goals: Focus on your career and professional aspirations. Set goals, continue to learn and grow in your field, and seek opportunities for advancement and fulfillment.

Remember, building a family is just one aspect of a fulfilling and purposeful life. Embrace the unique journey you are on, and know that there are many paths to finding happiness and fulfillment.

In conclusion, there are several key steps that individuals and couples can take to improve fertility and reduce the risk of miscarriage. These include maintaining a healthy lifestyle, managing stress levels, seeking medical assistance if necessary, and considering alternative therapies or treatments. It is crucial to remember that every individual and couple is unique, and what works for one may not work for another. Therefore, it is essential to consult with healthcare professionals to develop a personalized plan that addresses specific needs and factors influencing fertility and miscarriage risk. With proper care, support, and understanding, individuals and couples can increase their chances of conceiving and carrying a pregnancy to term.